SUR
MEDI

SURVIVALIST'S MEDICINE CHEST

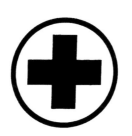

RAGNAR BENSON
PALADIN PRESS

Survivalist's Medicine Chest
by Ragnar Benson

Copyright © 1982 by Ragnar Benson

ISBN 13: 978-0-87364-256-9
Printed in the United States of America

Published by Paladin Press, a division of
Paladin Enterprises, Inc.
Gunbarrel Tech Center, 7077 Winchester Circle
Boulder, Colorado 80301 USA, +1.303.443.7250

Direct inquiries and/or orders to the above address.

Visit our website at www.paladin-press.com

WARNING

Neither the author nor publisher assumes any responsibility for the use or misuse of the information contained in this book. It is for emergency informational purposes only, and should be consulted only when a physician and/or conventional medical facilities are unavailable. Be warned!

Other books by Ragnar Benson:
Acquiring New ID
Do-It-Yourself Medicine
Eating Cheap
Guerrilla Gunsmithing
Live Off the Land in the City and Country
Mantrapping
Modern Survival Retreat
Modern Weapons Caching
Ragnar's Action Encyclopedias, Volumes 1 and 2
Ragnar's Guide to Interviews, Investigations, and Interrogations
Ragnar's Guide to the Underground Economy
Ragnar's Tall Tales
Ragnar's Ten Best Traps . . . And a Few Others That Are Damn Good, Too
Ragnar's Urban Survival
Starting a New Life in Rural America
Survival Nurse
Survival Poaching
Survival Retreat: A Total Plan for Retreat Defense

CONTENTS

INTRODUCTION

In the field of survivalist literature, there is no more commonly neglected topic than that of survival medicine. The reason behind this is not a lack of need or demand. I know from talking to folks around the country that there is a great hunger for new books of this type.

I've always thought there is a great irony here, in that you can find plenty of survival books about which guns and ammo to buy. But try and find a book on what to do after you get shot by the guns and ammo! They are mostly outdated military field manual reprints.

Anyway, it seems that the people who plan to survive through a government collapse or war realize one primary fact: that doctors and conventional medical facilities may become a luxury in the future. I know that it's a horribly grim concept to think about. But survivalists have never been afraid to face up to the idea of Doomsday. Wouldn't this simply amount to a hopeless future? I don't think so. Over the past forty years, I have often found myself in some of the most obscure and inhospitable regions on earth. Some places the natives had never seen a white man before. In others, the closest hospital was literally hundreds of miles away.

All of this didn't bother me as much as it might have bothered some folks, since I never went to see a regular doctor until I moved off our farm after I was eighteen. Mom and Dad couldn't afford to pay any doctor bills. It was that simple. So they made do the best way they could, in the finest spirit of American ingenuity: they doctored with veterinary medical supplies.

Which is what this book is all about.

Be assured that the vet medicines I will discuss are every bit as pure as their human counterparts. The only difference is the price. For instance, I know a druggist who orders both vet and human grades of tetracycline from the same pharmaceutical supply house. His orders for both are filled from the same batch of tetracycline. But the version of the drug with a vet-grade label costs much less than the human-label kind does—plus it can be purchased without a prescription.

Before I go any further, be warned that the procedures I present hereafter are to be used only during emergencies. Always consult a physician unless it is absolutely impossible to do so.

The *Survivalist's Medicine Chest* is not meant to be a one-stop source of comprehensive, do-it-yourself medical knowledge. It *is* a useful addition to any first-aid/emergency-medicine library, I believe. Books such as *Where There Is No Doctor, Medical Advisor's Handbook,* and *The Merck Manual* cover loads of topics that I will not touch on.

Yet I have no doubt that this effort is a worthwhile and valid adjunct to existing books on the subject. In the following pages, you will find advice on obtaining inexpensive supplies, how to diagnose common illnesses and injuries, and then how to treat them simply and efficiently. This knowledge has allowed me to save many lives over the years, including my own, on several hairy occasions.

I leave you with one parting thought, courtesy of Hippocrates, history's first great healer, who said: "Healing is a matter of time, but it is sometimes also a matter of opportunity."

A LESSON LEARNED

My Swahili was very patchy, but the message I was getting seemed to be of an emergency either recently past or impending. It was tough to tell which amongst all the excited babble. Apparently people I knew were involved, but other than that, I was at a loss to know exactly what was happening.

Without wasting any more time, I blew my whistle, alerting the members of my team as well as the work party. We had never gamed out a drill for the road workers, yet every time I blew my whistle, they wasted little time getting off the road into a hollow or depression where they could get hunkered down.

Below, I could see scattered rows of white eyes and white teeth shining up at me. To the right, perhaps four hundred yards, was my wife Kirsten. Within thirty seconds, silence settled on the area. The only noise was the sound of my two European friends running up the path toward me. Each carried an FN in one hand and a can of ammo in the other.

At the rondaavels I could see Kirsten crouching down behind the sandbag revetment. Every now and then, the large brass .375 rounds glinted in the sun. From where she was, Kirsten could cover three-fourths of the mountain saddle with her scoped Model 70. I had the high ground above, putting us in a pretty damn defensible position if trouble was on the way.

Two weeks earlier, we had been hit by Shifta irregulars at dawn. The raid had cost them five warriors. We lost an old woman, a young boy, and three warriors. This particular area in northern Kenya was the center of perpetual intertribal warfare. We would have been foolish not to react now as we were.

On seeing our response, the two old Samburu warriors realized that we were taking things damned seriously. One sat on the

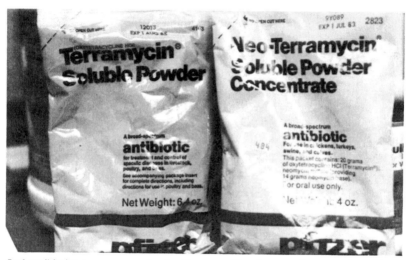

Oral antibiotics are necessary for treating everything from gunshot wounds to plague. Their packages are state-of-the-art in terms of shelf or refrigerator life, but the quantities are a problem, even in the smallest container. Consider breaking the 100 cc and 100 grain units into usable sizes while conditions are controlled.

ground, crossed his legs, and began babbling incoherently at the
dirt. The other took off like an antelope, his thin blue-black body
gyrating crazily as he ran down the green mountainside toward
the village. Within a couple of minutes, two Samburus started back
up the hill towards us. One, I could tell, was Ghedo, the only vil-
lager around who could really speak Swahili.

It took them an incredibly long time to make it back to where
the three of us stood. African bush natives, to the person, are in
poor physical condition. I never met one I couldn't outwalk or
outclimb. Now, back at the road, the three babbled on in Samburu
for several minutes. Finally Ghedo started in with the long awaited
explanation.

"Oh, Bwana," he said. "Remember that old woman who
brought you cedar wood for your stove in the rondaavel? The one
you liked so well?"—I hadn't beat or cursed her, so they assumed I
liked her.—"Well, she is dead up on the mountain."

"Dead!" I exclaimed. "How could that be? She was just here

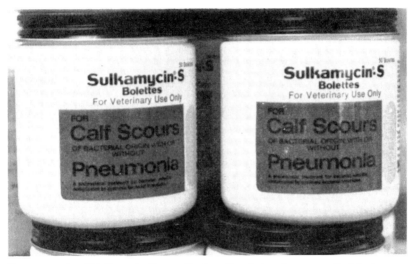

Common oral antibiotics and other medications identical to those prescribed for humans are available for pennies right off the farm dealer's shelves. But you have to learn to read the labels. This particular medication is a knock-out for diarrhea.

this morning showing me the new oryx-leather straps her husband made for her."

African husbands feel it is an act of kindness to give their wives heavy carrying straps. Then the women need make only half as many trips to haul their burdens and save all kinds of time and effort—or so goes the reasoning.

"Oh, Bwana," he answered, "she is not dead, but she will be dead very soon now. And she was such a valuable woman. It is all so bad!"

"Where is she?" I asked.

"Up on the mountain by the cedar trees where they left her," Ghedo replied. "She cut her foot with her ax and is dying."

Not only had I taken the time to look at the straps that morning, but in response to the old woman's request, I had sharpened her ax head on the grinder. The metal was nothing more than a piece of strap steel wound on a stick. Yet it was that instrument which cut up the wood we burned for heat and cooking that

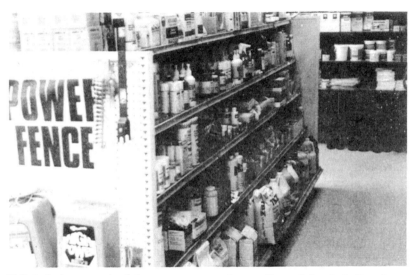

Well-stocked vet supply shelves are common wherever livestock is raised. Even internationally, many otherwise unavailable items can be purchased right off the shelf.

had apparently damaged the woman's foot.

Our policy in Africa was to provide medical assistance to all of the women who asked for it and to the men who worked for us or with us. Our obligation to the old woman was, therefore, clearly defined. I sent the three men up the hill to carry the woman down. They grumbled about the demeaning, disgusting nature of my request but dared not refuse. Paul went down to the dawa shack for the medical kit while I looked around for a clean patch of grass where I could work. We still weren't sure exactly what kind of emergency we faced, but apparently it would not entail any shooting.

Soon the three old buzzards returned with the woman. Without ceremony, they dumped her with a thud on the spot I pointed to. On examination we found that, although the wound would have been fatal for these people in their usual circumstances, it was not particularly serious given the bit of medical ability we possessed.

Apparently the ax had bounced off a branch and sliced open a slab of flesh on the side of her foot, starting about an inch behind her little toe and running to within about an inch of her heel. The cut did not go through the sole of her foot, but a thick flap of meat hung there grotesquely.

It appeared as though she had already lost a large quantity of blood. I prepared an antiseptic solution, washed the wound, and temporarily closed two small veins with hemostats. Meanwhile Kirsten gave her a shot to block the nerve below the knee. Neither of us had ever done the first hour of any kind of medical training. The thought of using a general anesthetic scared us, even though it might have been appropriate.

After cleaning out the wound a bit more and letting it dry for a minute, I dusted the cut with wound dressing powder and began to sew. Twenty-seven stitches later, the cut was closed. Our patient went into mild shock but otherwise seemed okay. We gave her 5 mg. of penicillin and a tetanus shot, bandaged the wound, and had her carried to a shade tree where she could spend a couple of days recovering.

There is no question in my mind that we saved the old gal's life. More important, in the context of this booklet, is the fact that every piece of equipment, every drop of medicine, and every bit of knowledge we used (and had been using for months to save people's lives) was originally intended for use in veterinary medicine. We didn't have the first ounce of anything made exclusively for humans.

Lest anyone think that this situation might be racist, let me point out that while I was growing up on the farm and until I was quite old, I never went to a doctor and never had any medication other than veterinary medical supplies. My grandparents used vet medicine as did my father. The only changes occurred as technology became more complex and we acquired antibiotics and sulfa drugs. Both my wife and I received all of our medical training and experience with animals. We learned to diagnose them, doctor them, sew them up, and vaccinate them. In so doing, we learned techniques that we later applied to doctoring each other.

The reason we went this route is fairly obvious to those folks who are inherently frugal or who were raised poor in a rural setting. Vet medical supplies are cheap, available without prescription, and are, from a sanitary-purity-safety standpoint, every bit as good as medication made for humans. In most cases, they are identical in composition. Only the labels have been changed, I believe.

But I realize that some people who read the following information are going to get themselves into trouble. The problem will not be with the medications, however, but with the poor techniques and inexperience of those using them. I guess the question here is the same one we faced in Africa. If the only help we can provide is based on veterinary supplies and information, are people who will die without medical attention better off left alone or helped by what we can provide?

My wife and I elected to help—both ourselves and the people

who became part of our group. Yet if you, the reader, know nothing about treating humans, pigs, horses, and cattle, you will sooner or later kill someone using the techniques in this booklet. Be sure you understand the consequences when you evaluate the trade-offs. The danger is not in the supplies, but in your having at your disposal supplies for which your skill levels are inadequate. Always keep this in mind as you read on through this information.

MEDICAL HARDWARE

Depending on where you live, you will probably have no difficulty locating ag supply houses that carry all of the vet medicine products I will mention. More of them exist in the smaller towns in the Middle West where great numbers of pigs, chickens, and cattle are raised, but I have always been able to find at least a few basic vet medications any place I have traveled—even in other countries.

Elevators, tack stores, feed stores, drug stores, equipment and supply outlets, and others that cater to farmers and ranchers carry vet medicines. Look in the Yellow Pages under "Veterinarian Equipment and Supplies" to find both retail and wholesale listings. Vet supplies are generally very inexpensive, but you may like

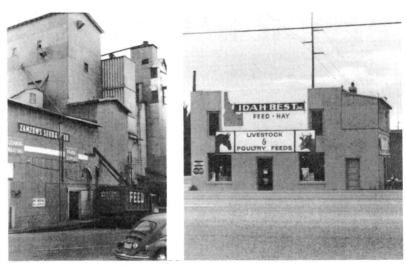

Large ag supply houses that are part of a feed mill complex often stock thousands of dollars worth of vet medical items. Almost any tiny farm store will stock some basic vet supplies. Both will order in the harder-to-get supplies that they don't normally carry.

to buy wholesale if you can. Often this is possible if you represent yourself as either being a veterinarian or having a retail store.

Most places don't do any background-checking on vets. I have called a huge number of suppliers who maintain that they sell only to licensed veterinarians, and by telling them—"This is Dr. Benson from an adjoining state and I am traveling through and would like to pick up some supplies."—I have always gotten what I wanted. If they ask for a license number or permit, tell them you don't remember but will have your girl call in the morning.

Some vet supplies are not traded on the open market. These require the equivalent of a prescription. Happily, there are very few of these, and they are mostly of limited utility for the survivor. Usually you can get around this prohibition by listing out a great number of items that are customarily traded on the open market in retail stores before coming around to the few that are narcotics or are otherwise restricted for some reason or another.

Disinfectants

One easily attainable and very important group of products to the survivor are the disinfectants. Solutions of this type are used to clean up treatment centers, equipment, and the victim.

Don't ever, *ever* forget that disinfectant techniques are the cornerstones of any medical program. All the sulfa and penicillin in the world can't overcome huge amounts of dirt and filth. The survivor must be an absolute nut on this issue.

All equipment must be thoroughly washed and then soaked in alcohol or, even better, in a solution of one of the multipurpose sanitizers and germicides. Syringes, especially if you use the reusable type, must be disassembled and soaked for no less than thirty minutes. If not that, they must be boiled for no less than thirty minutes in mildly rolling water. In most cases I do both.

Vet disinfectants are generally known as the "gentle iodine complexes." They come concentrated in gallon jugs and, depend-

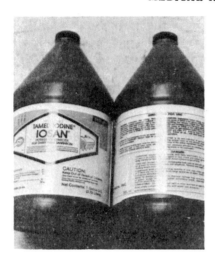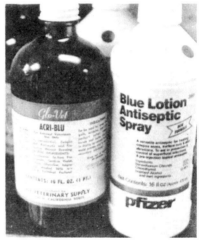

Disinfectants both for personal presurgical and sickroom cleanliness can be bought at farm supply stores. Some lack aesthetic considerations, however, as does this solution containing a dark-blue dye that lasts for weeks (left.)

ing on how you cut them with water, make good sickroom disinfectants or personal body disinfectants for use before and after minor surgery. Most larger vet supply stores carry or can order in denatured alcohol that also has practical application as a disinfectant.

Insecticides

Another extremely important product, especially for overseas use, are the insecticides. Available are many excellent, highly concentrated insecticides that can be used to spray living quarters. Or they can be applied directly to one's clothes and skin to keep malaria-carrying mosquitoes and plague-and typhus-carrying lice at bay. Good medical practice includes preventive measures and these insecticides help immensely. Most are Lindane based and should be diluted to one percent strength at most.

Syringes and Needles

Of the pieces of vet grade equipment needed by the survivor, probably none is more valuable than the syringe and needle. Two types are commonly available: the cheap, plastic throwaways and the more expensive stainless steel and glass models that can be disinfected and used over and over again. The problem with the reusables is that they must be thoroughly cleaned after each use. This is often difficult and time consuming.

When I had the medical detail in Cuba, Kenya, and India, I would line up my patients and give them a common dosage from a common syringe, changing only the needle. The plan worked well as long as there was a requirement for a production-line approach using the same antibiotic.

In Africa I ran the afternoon medical call for months where a lot of the Morani, or warriors, I treated had VD. It was far and away the most common malady they suffered. For five shillings, I gave them a three-shot series using vet grade procaine penicillin. I would line them up on a mark three feet from the dawa shack, have them drop their aprons, plant both palms on the wall, and

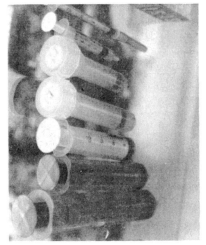 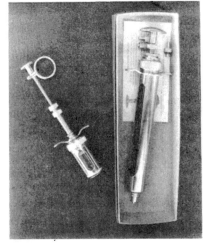

Throwaway syringes can be cleaned and sterilized for use a second and third time, if necessary. Reusable syringes with a dose meter (right) are often desirable. But clean-up is a problem. If not properly done, the dirty syringe can pose a horrible health hazard.

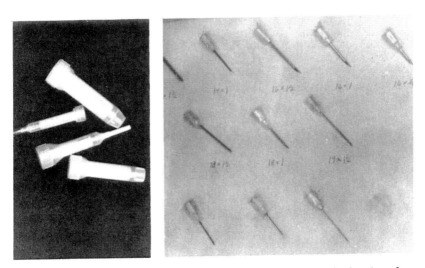

Plastic, disposable syringes (right) cost a few cents each and come in sizes from 2 cc to 60 cc. Injection needles are classified by size. The smaller, shorter sizes are best for using on humans.

then go down the line giving them each one dose. By slapping one on the ass, jamming in the needle, running the plunger to the stop, replacing the needle, slapping again, and going on to the next, I could do three or four a minute. I probably cured more VD in twelve months this way than most doctors see in a lifetime in this country.

Vet grade needles are sold by size as are those used in common medical practice. They run from number 14s through 22s or 24s. The higher the number, the smaller the diameter. Length is another criterion. You would, for instance, order a box of number 24s three-fourths of an inch long or perhaps number 20s two inches long for use on smaller hogs or people.

It would be nicer to buy smaller sizes for people, but this is seldom possible. I don't believe I have ever seen a vet grade needle less than number 24 being actually offered for sale. The larger sizes hurt a bit more and may occasionally leak back when heavy doses are given, but this is not an insurmountable problem. Some penicillin is so lumpy that large needles must be used. On the other hand, administering vaccines such as tetanus points up the need to have several syringes of various sizes. The doses of this and many other materials are very small and are tough to give using a 10 cc or larger syringe. Having a wide range of sizes of both needles and syringes is desirable.

Sewing Needles and Sutures

Other pieces of common hardware often of use to the survivor are the needles necessary to sew up cuts and wounds. As with the needles used on syringes, sewing needles come in sizes ranging from the horrible to the humane.

Generally I use number 13 through number 16, the smallest, on people. They also come in three-eighths circle or one-half circle. Deciding which ones to use depends on personal preference and the nature of the job at hand. All sewing needles are razor sharp and should be discarded after they have been used a time or two. Dull needles are the pits to work with.

Suture material is available in either black silk or dissolving-type gut. At times, unusually deep wounds must be sewed on several levels to close the breach correctly. You will want to use smaller dissolving sutures inside and close with larger black thread outside. When you do sew it up, be sure to close a cut in such a way that the wound can drain. I use common individually tied stitches and generally like to use many and keep them small, if possible.

Black thread is commonly available. Dissolving, internal suture material is a bit more difficult to come by. I have a fellow survivor friend who runs a farm supply store and orders in spools of the material for me. He has no problem obtaining the thread and any farm supply store should be willing to do likewise for you.

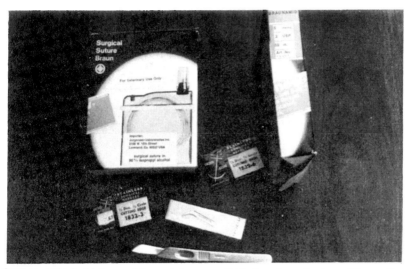

Sutures, scalpels, blades, and hemostats are available in vet supply stores. The smaller needles are suited for use on humans and must be held with a hemostat or needle holder.

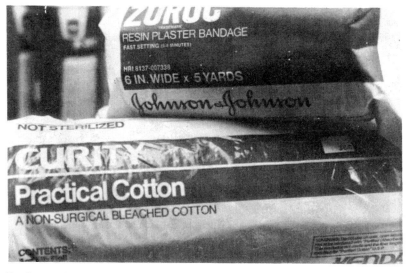

Bandages and prefab splint material is available over-the-counter or by special order.

Hemostats

Sewing needles without stainless steel hemostats to hold them are worthless. The needles are too small to hold in one's fingers, and, from contact, the wound becomes so dirty that it never heals. Besides that, hemostats are necessary for clamping blood vessels when performing minor surgery.

There are literally hundreds of kinds and sizes of hemostats. I have half a dozen of the five-inch models, both curved and straight-jawed, and a couple of three-inch models. It's best to go rummage through the dealer's supply to get what you need. You probably won't buy too many because they are relatively expensive. If you can find them, regular needle holders are available that work better than hemostats. Needles won't twist or turn in them, and some have a scissor combination built right in.

Scalpels

Another common piece of medical hardware is the scalpel.

These are stainless steel knives having thin, replaceable blades that are unusually sharp. In the animal husbandry business, these knives are used to castrate animals, so are readily available. There are three different styles of blades. Which you use is entirely a matter of personal preference.

Intravenous Sets

If you consider yourself well trained and believe you will want to handle giving intravenous solutions, you may want to buy an infusion set. Vet models are basically the same as those made to be used on humans and are safe in the proper hands. Of course, if you don't know what you are doing, you will kill somebody using this gear.

The set comes in a storage bag and includes the tubing and flow monitor. Then, all that is needed are the intravenous needle sets to go with the rest of the outfit. Administering a general anesthetic, electrolytes, or other solutions will require your having an

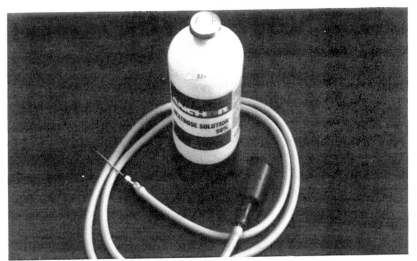

Intravenous devices are used in vet medicine. This simple outfit might work in an emergency, but if you expect to give general anesthetics, you will need a model that has flow metering and valves.

infusion set. Happily, they are about half the price of regular medical models. Livestock dextrose solution may be given intravenously in an emergency situation. It is identical to some of the solutions used for humans.

Splints

Although they are not yet common in most farm supply stores, a very nice line of lightweight splints is available to veterinarians. Many times, even in this day and age, an animal that suffers a broken leg is destroyed, explaining why prefab splints are not common. They can be ordered in and make excellent devices for the survivor.

Cat-size splints work on fingers, dog-size fit most arms, and pig-size are suitable for legs. If these prefab splints are not available, there is always the old gauze and plaster of Paris method of making a cast for the broken limb. So far, though, the farm store purchasing managers have always been more than willing to get splints for me.

DIAGNOSIS
AND TREATMENT

Before starting on a situation-by-situation look at using vet grade medicines for doctoring humans, the survivor should realize an important cornerstone fact. Of all the mammals roving the earth, none are more similar to humans in many, many regards than pigs are. It is my understanding that no animal's digestive needs, for instance, are more humanlike than a pig's. Not even primates require a diet more similar to a man's than the common hog.

Because this is true, the survivor can look at the dosages recommended for hogs on the various bottles of antibiotics, figure the dosage for a person according to his body weight, and get a reasonable approximation of how much medicine to administer.

Keep this in mind when evaluting all vet medicines, *both internal and external.*

As a general rule, animals are treated on the basis of body weight. Most livestockmen are aware of, but do not use, antibiotics on the basis of the number of units they contain per cubic centimeter. In other words, they look at the bottle to be sure they are getting a fairly high concentration of medication for their money, but when they treat, they look at the recommendation for a specific animal according to estimated body weight. When treating humans, it is definitely the better part of wisdom to look up the *exact* recommended dosage in units and treat with that on the suggested time schedule.

Treatment of gas gangrene, for instance, requires that two million units of penicillin be given every three hours. In the case of anthrax, the book suggests giving ten million units daily. Some medications are prescribed on the basis of milligrams per kilogram of body weight. This should present little problem to the knowl-

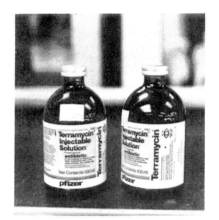 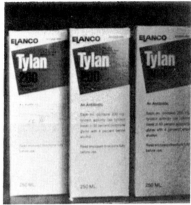

Vet medical supplies are relatively inexpensive. These 100 cc bottles of Terramycin will treat pneumonia and plague and cost under $3 each. The problem lies with amateurs who don't know what they are doing. The Tylan is a powerful drug not considered safe for humans.

edgeable technician. Read the label on the bottle and a good medical book before starting in.

I would suggest that if you are going to play doctor and take someone's life in your hands, you get a copy of *Current Medical Diagnosis and Treatment* edited by Marcus Krupp and Milton Chatton. It is available from the publisher, Lange Medical Publications, Drawer L, Los Altos, CA, 94022. The 1983 version costs twenty-five dollars and is worth every penny. Obviously this is not the only medical book the survivor should own, but it is the most valuable one when interfacing vet medical supplies with materials used by doctors.

Burns

In a third world context, the most common malady I treated was VD. But in a strictly paramilitary situation, I guess burns caused me the most grief. Looking at burns first, there are several excellent vet products one can usually buy off the shelf—depending on the location and stock the dealer commits to carrying—that contain either silver sulfadiazine or mafenide. The trade names are Silvadene and Sulfamylon, respectively. Both are miracle-class burn products that are disgustingly expensive outside an ag context.

These medicines come as salves that are smeared on the burn. Consult the label for exact instructions. Usually the stuff is stronger than needed for doctoring people and must be put on sparingly or diluted. The burn is left open or lightly bandaged when treated with Silvadene or Sulfamylon. The only purpose for the covering is to keep out dirt and contamination.

Dimethyl Sulfoxide (DMSO) is used extensively to treat horses. It is a carrier that will bring medication into a foal while it is still being carried by a mare. Much has been written about DMSO lately. Personally, I am leary of the stuff because of its ability to carry toxic materials into the body. Nevertheless, I have seen it work very well to treat burns. You can buy it by the liter off your vet supplier's shelf for a fraction of the cost a drugstore sells it for.

Bad burns always carry with them a danger of infection, so a shot of penicillin may be necessary if infections set in. Procaine penicillin is generally the medication of choice. Of all the vet products available, the broad spectrum antibiotics are the most useful and the most abundant. Virtually every little ag supply store has a refrigerator with a supply of 50 or 100 cc bottles of penicillin in it.

Venereal Disease

Internationally, the most common use of penicillin seems to be to treat gonorrhea. I passed out literally hundreds of liters of the stuff in Asia and Africa. My greatest problem was getting the diseased to come back for their second and third shots. As soon as they felt better, they would often take off for the bush, only to return a month or two later with a much more difficult, much more resistant variety of crotch rot. Wherever I have been, gonor-

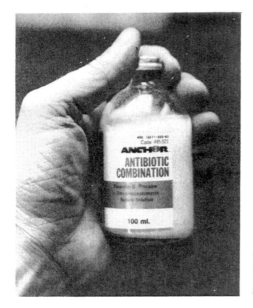

Combiotic, containing penicillin and sulfa drugs, is the old stand-by for farmers. It currently sells for about $2.50 for a 100 cc bottle.

rhea has been the venereal disease of the masses, but the treatment for syphillis is identical.

Assuming you are not treating a resistant variety, the antibiotic that is easiest to acquire and use is either penicillin G Procaine or penicillin G Benzathine. Both are available in 10, 25, 50, 100 and 250 cc vials from virtually every ag supply store refrigerator. The cost is so low you will not believe it. Often a 250 cc bottle can be purchased for under six dollars.

Unless you plan to run some sort of field hospital, stick with buying the smaller bottles. By being careful, it is possible to remove 5 ccs at a time from a 250 cc bottle, but the technique is tough and easily compromised. Penicillin is used in massive doses in the animal-raising industry to combat shipping fever, foot rot, diptheria, wound infections, pneumonia, and a host of other bacterial diseases. It is often given 20 ccs at a time to dozens of critters, explaining why such large bottles are commonly available.

Humans are usually best off if given *procaine* penicillin of

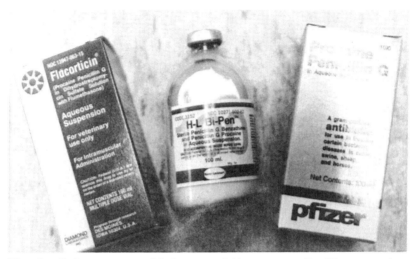

Virtually all the common antibiotics are available as vet supplies. These are various brands of Procaine G penicillin.

some sort if it is available. Procaine is a pain killer. Raw penicillin stings mightily when injected into a muscle. The combination of the two makes things go a whole lot smoother and with far less pain. More about pain killers later.

Should you run into a tough, resistant strain of VD that does not respond to penicillin, or if you know from past experience that your patient can't handle penicillin, try oral tetracycline. This material is available in tablet form for use in fighting calf scours (diarrhea). The dosage from a single pill is way too large for humans. Depending on the label, you will have to cut it down by one-third or one-fourth. Tetracycline is also available as an injectable. Treatment of choice is a matter of preference on the part of the medic. I believe it is wise to have both materials available since neither requires much money or storage space.

Anyone who gives shots of any kind must be prepared to handle a shock condition known as *anaphylaxis* which is an allergic reaction to the injected material. Death can occur in as little as ten minutes, requiring that one immediately know what is happening and why. Animals are no different than people in this regard. Anyone who engages in the practice of vet medicine always has a bottle of epinephrine handy which is an adrenal hormone stimulant. It is commonly available in all vet medicine supply stores under that name.

To make things go smoothly in an emergency situation, I pump my epinephrine bottle full of air using a sterile syringe and needle. Hold the bottle upside down and run the air through the liquid. When you need a dose in a hurry, simply insert the needle back into the bottle and allow the pressure to blow the syringe full. This technique works for any injectable, even if you are not in any particular rush.

As with any shock situation, have your patient lie down, put his feet up, keep warm, and, if possible, block or remove the cause of the pain.

Pneumonia

Although I have never had much problem with it, pneumonia is the bane of many people in a paramilitary or survival situation. This is especially true in the more northern climates. As with VD, the patient should respond well to either of the penicillins or, that failing, to tetracycline.

Diarrhea

One of the really great scourges I faced on overseas assignments was diarrhea. There were times when I desperately needed to be out patrolling but instead had to sit under some godforsaken tree pooping my guts out. Often my native workers caught something or other and were similarly indisposed. This was especially true in southeast Asia.

Some diarrhea is directly traceable to a major problem such as cholera, plague, or the like. Most, however, is simply caused by a low-grade bacterial infection from drinking the water, eating un-

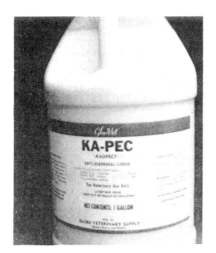 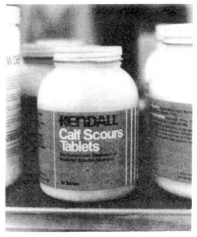

Nonprescription vet medicines are often much more concentrated than drugs for humans and cost a fraction of their price. Do you recognize this treatment for diarrhea (left). Calves and piglets frequently suffer from diarrhea and are given "calf scours" tablets. Just be sure to cut the medication for human use.

cooked vegetables or dirty fruit, or lacking in general sanitation. In many, many cases, there is the chicken and the egg syndrome wherein diet and vitamin loss contribute to the overall problem. Happily, the same thing happens to animals—particularly calves and piglets. A dynamite vet product exists that combines neomycin with vitamins and minerals in an incredibly concentrated form that has *always* worked for me to control the runs. It is known as "calf and pig scours powder." Just be double sure you cut the dose way down. The stuff is really concentrated.

Another product can also be used for serious bacterial enteritis and is especially useful when the patient is so far gone that oral treatment may not be practical. Generally it should be used along with intravenous solutions, putting it in the class of serious medication that is used only as a last resort. The product is known as oxytetracycline (HCl), and the trade names are Oxytet 50, Oxytet 100, and Terramycin. There are usually two densities or strengths. On humans, I always use the milder Oxytet 50.

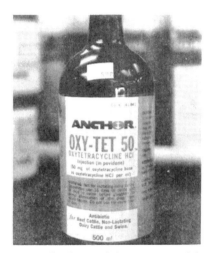
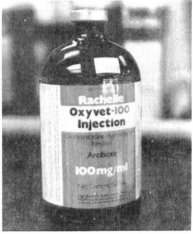

Tetracycline is one of the most powerful, general-purpose antibiotics available. It treats everything from infected wounds to VD and anthrax. Oxy-tet 50 can also be used to treat humans, but be sure you read directions first.

As I mentioned earlier, tetracycline is also extensively used to handle problems that cannot be cleared up with penicillin or for patients who might react unfavorably to regular antibiotics. The field medic has an incredible array of products available to him off the vet supply shelf—so many that they can become confusing if his grounding in the general area of medicines and medical techniques is not sound. Because scours (bacterial diarrhea) is so common to livestock, there exists a wide range of products to treat it. Thoroughly peruse your dealer's shelf before you buy.

Eye Infections

Eye infections and eye injuries requiring more than simple boric acid treatments are other common medical problems that the survivor and paramilitary medic face. Some eye maladies are extremely complex and difficult to handle which is why there is specialization in this area within the medical profession. However, in probably 80 percent of the cases, the survivor will be concerned

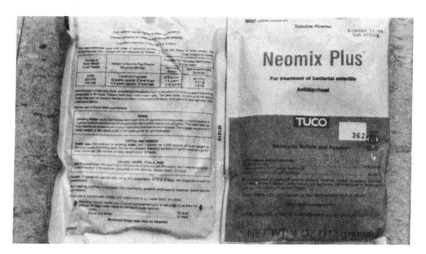

Some drugs are similar to, but not the same as, drugs used for humans. A good working knowledge of these and a good reference book are necessary. *Physician's Desk Reference,* published by Medical Economics Company, is invaluable for cross-checking possible medications.

with either remedying acute bacterial infection or controlling bacterial infection after an injury has occurred. These can be nicely treated with a group of vet products used to handle mastitis or udder infections in cattle.

The recommended procedure is to dose with either a broad spectrum antibiotic or medications in the sulfonamide group. These are available as a procaine penicillin salve or as a tri-sulfa solution. A tri-sulfa solution contains three sulfa drugs; three common ones are sulfapyridine, sulfamethazine and sulfathiazole. In its stock form, it is usually about 12 percent concentration, meaning it should be cut about five times before being used. The same is true with the antibiotic salves: they should be cut with Vaseline by at least four to one before they are used. Consult the label directions and the medical books before wildly rushing off to treat eyes. In this case, be absolutely *sure* you are the remedy of last resort.

Eye problems are generally much more painful than other injuries. Most of the topical ointments containing penicillin also contain procaine. For that reason, I tend to like to use that medication. It keeps the injured from suffering so much without anesthetizing the eye so thoroughly that it becomes a danger to the patient.

Pinkeye medications can also be of value in treating eye infections but are generally not suitable for human use. The granules tend to be too large and coarse. In an emergency, one could make them into a paste, but generally it is better to stay with the mastitis remedies. Pinkeye medicines are best used in treating open cuts.

Wounds

When sewing up a wound, one of the best materials in the world—bar none—to promote healing and ease pain is the pinkeye powder originally intended for cattle. The medication has sulfa, an antiseptic, an antibiotic, and an anesthetic in it. The only pre-

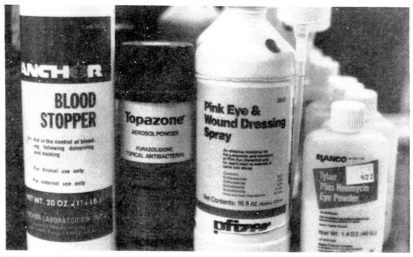

Pinkeye medications, which work wonders in healing wounds, are examples of vet medicines that have uses not entirely obvious. They contain antiseptics, antibiotics, and an anesthetic. Blood coagulant may be useful in treating wounds, too.

caution is *don't ever use it heavily*. It is a wonderful medicine, but if the wound is packed with the stuff, the body will reject the whole mess, creating a festering, nasty sore. Dust it on lightly and call it good.

Blood coagulant may be helpful when used on serious wounds that do not involve an artery or major vein. Mostly, though, compresses held directly on the wound will stop bleeding.

General infection from a nonspecific source such as bullet or stabbing wounds, are treated with penicillin G Benzathine. The wound may be opened with a scalpel and drained, then cleaned with disinfectants. Treat it with pinkeye powder and stitch it closed.

Tetanus

Puncture wounds carry with them the danger of lockjaw or tetanus. Virtually all Americans have been vaccinated for immunity, but many foreign nationals have not. Depending on the recommended dosage listed on the bottle, I give .5 cc of tetanus *antitoxin* as a booster when treating a patient who has a puncture wound or cut. If you have the time, you might want to immunize your entire crew of foreign nationals using tetanus *toxoid* if they have not been previously immunized. Both injectable products are easily available out of your animal health products dealer's refrigerator.

Internal Parasites

Another readily available vet product that has more general application overseas than in this country, at least at present, are the internal wormers. I used gallons of piperazine on the men in Africa with very good results.

In warm climates, internal parasites proliferate mightily, sapping the people's energy as well as the utility of the food they eat. Piperazine gets all the major critters except hookworms and tapeworms. Several good wormers for use on these pests are avail-

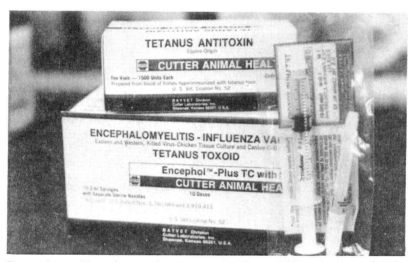

Tetanus is a problem whenever there are wounds. The toxoid is used to immunize, the antitoxin is given as a booster when the wound is treated. Premeasured doses of these are available but are too large for humans. Read the labels.

able over-the-counter in other countries. They are not offered in the United States even to M.D.s.

Low Energy

When pepping up villagers, the other half of the equation consists of proper diet. In Africa where the dietary requirements under normal circumstances are virtually never met, this is especially important. I could *always* tell when I was dealing with Africans who were raised in a mission school, for instance. On the average, they were six inches taller and thirty pounds heavier than other bush natives from the same tribe.

Animal vitamin and mineral premix packages provide a nice inexpensive resolution to the problem of raising the nutritional standard of people. There are also excellent injectable vitamin A-D-B$_{12}$ products for use on dangerously malnourished, debilitated patients. Injectable iron can help when a person suffers from anemia. Read the label and administer the dosage for hogs of the same weight. Results are often dramatic.

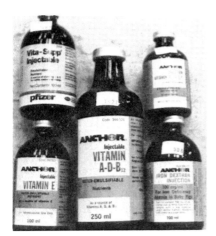 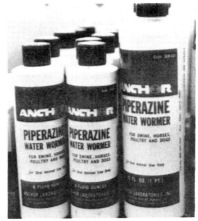

Injectable vitamins (right) are useful for treatment of diarrhea and poor nutrition. When dealing with noncritical health products, use dosage recommended for hogs of the same weight. Common internal parasites can be treated with piperazine in both animals and humans.

Pain

Handling pain in the sick and injured is tough for the survivor. The pain-killers sodium pentothal, chloroform, and procaine are all available from vet supply houses. Of these three, procaine is the easiest for the layman to acquire. None of these materials are available right off the shelf, unlike everything else mentioned up to this point. You might be able to buffalo your way past the clerk at a vet medicine supply house, have a survival-oriented vet order it for you, or get a sympathetic farm supply store manager to sell you some of the common pain killer. But since distribution of these drugs is closely controlled, no matter which route you take, it won't be easy.

I dislike, and am afraid of, administering general anesthetics using materials such as sodium pentothal. If you must do it to set bones or sew up a bad abdominal wound, then so be it. Just pray that you have had some instruction in the use of these materials before you are called on to do the job.

Sodium pentothal is administered intravenously in fairly large doses. Putting the stuff in the patient is no real problem. General intravenous vet equipment, as I pointed out, is available. The trick is getting the dosage right—not too little, not too much. There are charts and graphs you can use to determine dosage based on body weight, but there still must be a great sensitivity to the general vital signs of the patient.

Chloroform is not a good general anesthetic. It is dangerous and can, at best, easily cause pneumonia. On the other hand, it is usually pretty easy to buy. For that reason I have used it on animals quite a few times. I have also killed quite a few animals with chloroform. It is tough to determine when the patient is properly anesthetized and when you have gone over the deep end and given too much.

When I was a kid, I had a pet badger that I kept around the house for a couple of years. It was reasonably tame and got along well with our family. A friend I often played with talked me into letting him take my badger home to show his folks. In the strange surroundings, the little critter panicked and ran into the living room behind the couch. Their big German shepherd tried to nab it and was thoroughly bloodied by the badger. When I got there, the living room was a mess. They had all the doors shut tight and were trying to get the wounds on the dog's throat and neck closed.

My friend's old man gave me a bottle of chloroform to subdue my, by now, wild pet. I tore a gunny sack in half and liberally sprinkled the cloth with chloroform. As I advanced, my badger jumped out at me. I stuck the cloth ball in its face and let it bite down. It almost gassed me, but eventually the badger went limp, and I was able to fully cover its nose and mouth. I threw the rag in the saddlebag of my motor bike, along with the badger, and headed home. But, alas, I had done the job too well. The badger never recovered. I still have the skin on the wall.

Procaine is the pain killer I now use almost exclusively. With a long, slim needle, I can do a fairly credible job blocking nerves in the extremities. This allows me to sew or set without causing the patient to pass out from pain.

As I said before, this is a tough area. Be sure you know what you are doing, or that it is a life and death situation if you don't do something.

Skin Infections

Skin infections, including maladies caused by fungus such as athlete's foot, are bothersome, especially in the tropics. Before you begin treatment, be sure you are not dealing with anthrax or burns. If not, treat with one of the vet solutions made for fungal disorders. Look for those containing iodine or, better yet, potassium permanganate. There are a number of products on the market made to treat skin disorders in barnyard animals.

Rashes and some fungus-caused disorders can be dried with

alcohol and dusted with cornstarch. This is an old farmer's trick that works well except for stubborn skin problems that require zinc oxide or antibiotic ointments.

Another common, almost-forgotten farm cure is the use of Bag Balm on minor cuts and scrapes. The stuff is absolutely miraculous in its ability to promote healing. It was developed long, long ago to treat chapped teats on cows, horses, and pigs. Just rub a small amount on the minor wound.

Muscle Aches

Absorbine rub was originally developed for horses. It is a good product for muscle fatigue and sprain when used sparingly or diluted with alcohol.

Anthrax

When I first went to Africa, I ran into a number of people with burnlike wounds that festered and refused to heal. I treated

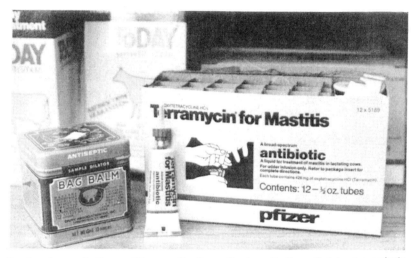

Be alert for survival/paramilitary applications of vet medications that treat seemingly unrelated maladies. Mastitis remedies are useful for eye infections and Bag Balm works wonders on minor cuts and scrapes.

their sores as I would have treated burns, which was all right, although I was not, as it turned out, dealing with burns. I used penicillin G and/or tetracycline for what I found out was anthrax.

It is my belief that North American survivors will see more and more of this stuff. It lives forever in the soil and occurs when personal sanitary standards fall. There is a common vet grade vaccination for anthrax, but I believe it is pretty rough on humans.

Tularemia

Another disease that will almost certainly proliferate is tularemia. It is spread by handling infected animals, particularly rabbits and muskrats, two critters that will be used as a food source by survivors. Treatment is drastic. Use streptomycin intramuscularly in combination with tetracycline orally.

Gangrene

Paramilitary contenders populating war zones often face horrible gangrene problems. In a warm climate, small wounds can quickly degenerate into blood poisoning and gangrene leading to the extremely unpleasant and difficult choice for the layman of either amputating the limb or letting the wounded person die.

At the first signs of problems, use massive doses of penicillin as prescribed by your medical manuals. Also, start right in with a tetanus series as previously described.

Brucellosis

Another serious malady that increases dramatically among rural people with little or no access to modern medical and sanitary facilities is brucellosis, also called Mediterranean or undulant fever. It is my belief that we will see lots of this stuff in years to come. The best prevention is to be careful not to drink unpasteurized milk or handle infected meat. That failing, treat with the good old stand-bys, tetracycline and streptomycin.

Animal Bites

Animal bites that become infected can be treated with oral and injectable antibiotics and sulfa powders and cleaned with animal grade disinfectants. Vet grade rabies vaccines exist, but I have never had to use them.

Typhoid fever

There is no vet grade immunization material that I know of available for typhoid fever, yet a person engaged in paramilitary operations for extended periods of time will almost certainly run into this crud. Most Americans going overseas have been immunized for it, but many foreign nationals have not. Whenever sanitation facilities break down and the water supply is contaminated, look for typhoid fever to occur.

In the context of typhoid fever is a good place to mention the drug ampicillin. It is about the only thing available that works on

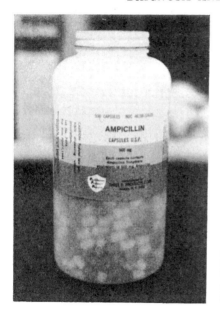

Ampicillin is one of the few drugs that works to cure typhoid fever, a Third World illness linked with dirty drinking water. But due to its potency, it is easily misused by the unaware.

typhoid fever. Fortunately it is a common vet product and is reasonably priced. The material keeps well and should be part of every survivor's medical kit. This drug should, because of its potency, be used carefully. Its application can be very broad among the resistant bacterial disorders.

Strep throat

Streptococcal throat infections sometimes spread like wildfire through groups of persons living in cold, meager conditions. Good old reliable penicillin G Benzathine knocks this bug nicely.

CONCLUSION

Obviously the list of common problems that can be success-fully treated with common vet grade medicines could fill a large book. On the other hand, it is probably equally apparent to the reader that most of the diseases, sicknesses, accidents, and condi-tions are best treated by a few common materials in the antibiotic and sulfa drug class.

Gunshot wounds, cuts, and punctures that would otherwise be fatal in a paramilitary or survival situation can be handled using a handful of vet products bought right off the shelf for fif-teen dollars or less. As a practical matter, the fifteen bucks would probably buy enough medical supplies for fifteen or twenty people!

This fact should be a great source of comfort for those who will be with you. For the price of a 50 cc bottle of injectable penicillin, a disposable syringe or two (which can, by the way, be cleaned up and used again), some wound dressing, sewing needles, a scalpel, sutures, and a few oral antibiotics, you can put together a kit that will save your people from dying from probably 60 percent of the wounds they are likely to suffer. Otherwise, most of these would be horrible, painful, and probably fatal.

My point, which I have made over and over, is that a fairly large group of common human maladies can be successfully treated with a relatively small family of readily available veterinarian products. If the medial problems are more complex, it will take a doctor to diagnose them anyway. And a doctor will more than likely have the exotic materials needed to handle the job.

In the meantime, remember that, while using vet medicines is a safe, easy way of handling medical situations, the burden of responsibility is still on the user. If you don't know what you are

doing and still insist on fooling around with the materials as out-
lined in this booklet, you will kill someone. It's that simple.